Nutrition
Essentials

A Beginner's Guide to Vital Nutrients

CONTENTS

INTRODUCTION

INTRODUCTION

The human body requires a wide range of nutrients to function properly and maintain good health. These nutrients can be divided into several categories, including:

MACRONUTRIENTS:
CARBOHYDRATES:

Provide energy and are found in foods like grains, fruits, vegetables, and legumes.

PROTEINS:

Essential for growth, repair, and maintenance of body tissues. Sources include meat, fish, eggs, dairy, and plant-based options like beans and tofu.

FATS (LIPIDS):

Provide energy, support cell growth, and are crucial for absorbing fat-soluble vitamins. Found in oils, nuts, seeds, and fatty fish.

MICRONUTRIENTS:
VITAMINS:

Organic compounds necessary for various biochemical processes. Examples include vitamin A, C, D, E, and K, as well as various B vitamins.

MINERALS:

Inorganic elements essential for various bodily functions. Examples include calcium, magnesium, potassium, sodium, iron, zinc, and selenium.

WATER:

Vital for hydration, temperature regulation, digestion, and various biochemical reactions. It's essential for overall health.

FIBER:

A type of carbohydrate found in plant foods like fruits, vegetables, whole grains, and legumes. It supports digestive health and helps prevent constipation.

ANTIOXIDANTS:

Compounds like vitamins C and E, beta-carotene, and selenium that help protect cells from damage caused by free radicals.

PHYTONUTRIENTS:

Bioactive compounds found in plants that have health-promoting properties. Examples include flavonoids, polyphenols, and phytochemicals.

ESSENTIAL FATTY ACIDS:

Omega-3 and omega-6 fatty acids are essential for brain function, reducing inflammation, and maintaining healthy skin and hair. They are found in fatty fish, nuts, and seeds.

AMINO ACIDS:

The building blocks of proteins, some of which are essential, meaning they must be obtained through the diet. Examples include leucine, lysine, and tryptophan.

ELECTROLYTES:

Minerals like sodium, potassium, calcium, and magnesium are critical for nerve function, muscle contraction, and maintaining fluid balance.

CHOLINE:

An essential nutrient that plays a role in various bodily processes, including brain health and liver function. It's found in foods like eggs, liver, and soybeans.

TRACE ELEMENTS:

Minerals like iodine (important for thyroid function), copper, manganese, and molybdenum that are needed in small amounts.

PROBIOTICS:

Beneficial bacteria that support gut health and digestion when consumed in foods like yogurt or taken as supplements.

A balanced diet that includes a variety of foods from different food groups ensures that the body receives all these essential nutrients. Nutritional needs can vary based on age, sex, activity level, and specific health conditions, so it's important to tailor your diet accordingly and, if needed, consult a healthcare professional or registered dietitian for personalized guidance.

MACRONUTRIENTS

MACRONUTRIENTS

Macronutrients are the essential nutrients that make up the bulk of the calories in your diet and provide your body with the energy it needs to function properly. There are three primary macronutrients:

CARBOHYDRATES:

Carbohydrates are a primary source of energy for the body. They are broken down into glucose, which can be used for immediate energy or stored as glycogen in the muscles and liver for later use. Good sources of carbohydrates include grains (e.g., rice, wheat, oats), fruits, vegetables, legumes, and sugary foods.

PROTEINS:

Proteins are essential for building and repairing tissues in the body. They are made up of amino acids, which are the building blocks of the body. Protein-rich foods include meat, poultry, fish, eggs, dairy products, legumes, nuts, and seeds.

FATS:

Dietary fats are important for energy storage, insulation, and the absorption of fat-soluble vitamins (A, D, E, and K). Healthy sources of dietary fats include avocados, nuts, seeds, olive oil, fatty fish (e.g., salmon, mackerel), and some dairy products. It's important to choose healthy fats, such as unsaturated fats, while limiting saturated and trans fats.

The proportion of these macronutrients in your diet can vary based on your individual needs and goals. For instance, athletes and individuals with certain medical conditions may have different macronutrient requirements. It's essential to maintain a balanced diet that provides an adequate intake of all three macronutrients to support overall health and well-being.

MICRONUTRIENTS

MICRONUTRIENTS

Micronutrients are essential nutrients that the body requires in smaller quantities compared to macronutrients (carbohydrates, proteins, and fats). Despite their lower calorie contribution, micronutrients play crucial roles in various physiological processes and are necessary for overall health. The primary micronutrients include:

VITAMINS:

These are organic compounds that serve as coenzymes or cofactors in various biochemical reactions in the body. There are two main categories of vitamins:

FAT-SOLUBLE VITAMINS:

These include vitamins A, D, E, and K. They are soluble in fats and are stored in the body's fatty tissues. Sources of fat-soluble vitamins include liver, dairy products, leafy greens, and certain oils.

WATER-SOLUBLE VITAMINS:

These include the B-complex vitamins (e.g., B1, B2, B3, B6, B12, folate) and vitamin C. They dissolve in water and are not stored in the body to the same extent as fat-soluble vitamins. Good sources of water-soluble vitamins include fruits, vegetables, whole grains, and lean proteins.

MINERALS:

These are inorganic substances that are essential for various physiological functions, such as bone health, nerve function, and fluid balance. Important minerals include calcium, potassium, sodium, magnesium, phosphorus, iron, zinc, selenium, and others. Mineral-rich foods include dairy products, leafy greens, nuts, seeds, and lean meats.

TRACE ELEMENTS:

Some micronutrients are required in trace amounts but are still essential for health. These include iodine (important for thyroid function), copper, manganese, molybdenum, and chromium. These trace elements are found in various foods but are generally required in very small quantities.

Micronutrient deficiencies can lead to various health problems and diseases. To maintain optimal health, it's important to consume a balanced diet that includes a variety of foods rich in vitamins, minerals, and trace elements. In some cases, dietary supplements may be recommended to address specific deficiencies or health conditions, but it's generally best to obtain micronutrients from a diverse and well-rounded diet.

WATER

WATER

Water is one of the most critical and fundamental substances for life. It plays numerous essential roles in the human body and is vital for maintaining overall health and well-being. Here are some key aspects of water:

HYDRATION:

Water is essential for maintaining proper hydration in the body. It helps regulate body temperature, transport nutrients and oxygen to cells, remove waste products, and support various metabolic processes.

CELLULAR FUNCTION:

Water is a major component of cells and is involved in virtually all cellular processes. It acts as a solvent, allowing chemical reactions to take place within cells.

DIGESTION:

Water is necessary for the proper functioning of the digestive system. It helps break down food in the stomach and intestines, facilitates the absorption of nutrients, and aids in the elimination of waste through bowel movements.

CIRCULATION:

Blood is primarily composed of water. Adequate hydration is essential for maintaining blood volume and circulation, which, in turn, supports the delivery of oxygen and nutrients to body tissues.

TEMPERATURE REGULATION:

Sweating is the body's natural cooling mechanism, and it relies on water to regulate body temperature. When you're overheated, you sweat to release excess heat, and evaporation of sweat helps cool the body.

JOINT LUBRICATION:

Water provides lubrication to joints, helping to reduce friction and prevent joint pain and stiffness.

DETOXIFICATION:

The kidneys rely on water to filter waste products and toxins from the blood, which are then excreted as urine.

It's important to maintain proper hydration by drinking an adequate amount of water each day. The daily water needs can vary based on factors such as age, sex, activity level, and climate, but a general guideline is to aim for around 8 glasses (64 ounces) of water per day for most adults. However, individual hydration needs may vary, and it's essential to listen to your body's signals for thirst.

Remember that other beverages and foods also contribute to your daily water intake. Fruits and vegetables, for example, have high water content and can contribute significantly to your hydration. Staying adequately hydrated is crucial for overall health, energy levels, and the proper functioning of bodily systems.

FIBER

FIBER

Fiber is a type of carbohydrate found in plant-based foods that the human body cannot digest or absorb. Instead of being broken down and absorbed, fiber passes relatively intact through the digestive system. There are two main types of dietary fiber:

SOLUBLE FIBER:

This type of fiber dissolves in water to form a gel-like substance. It can help lower blood cholesterol levels and stabilize blood sugar levels. Foods rich in soluble fiber include oats, barley, beans, lentils, fruits (especially citrus fruits), and some vegetables (like Brussels sprouts).

INSOLUBLE FIBER:

Insoluble fiber does not dissolve in water and adds bulk to the stool. It helps prevent constipation and promotes regular bowel movements by speeding up the passage of food and waste through the digestive tract. Foods rich in insoluble fiber include whole grains, wheat bran, nuts, seeds, and many vegetables (such as broccoli and carrots).

Fiber offers several important health benefits:

DIGESTIVE HEALTH:

Insoluble fiber helps prevent constipation by adding bulk to the stool and promoting regular bowel movements. Soluble fiber can help alleviate diarrhea by absorbing excess water in the digestive tract.

HEART HEALTH:

Soluble fiber can lower LDL (bad) cholesterol levels in the blood, reducing the risk of heart disease. It may also help lower blood pressure and inflammation.

BLOOD SUGAR CONTROL:

Soluble fiber can slow the absorption of sugar, helping to stabilize blood sugar levels. This is particularly beneficial for individuals with diabetes or those at risk of developing diabetes.

WEIGHT MANAGEMENT:

High-fiber foods tend to be filling and can help control appetite, which can aid in weight management by reducing overall calorie intake.

GUT HEALTH:

Fiber serves as food for beneficial gut bacteria, promoting a healthy gut microbiome. A diverse and healthy gut microbiome is associated with various health benefits.

To incorporate more fiber into your diet, consider the following:

- Choose whole grains over refined grains (e.g., whole wheat bread instead of white bread).
- Eat plenty of fruits and vegetables, including the skin when appropriate.
- Include legumes (beans, lentils, and peas) in your meals.
- Snack on nuts and seeds.
- Gradually increase your fiber intake to avoid digestive discomfort.

It's important to drink plenty of water when increasing your fiber intake to prevent potential digestive issues. Overall, a diet rich in fiber can contribute to better digestive health, heart health, and overall well-being.

ANTIOXIDANTS

ANTIOXIDANTS

Antioxidants are molecules that help protect the body from harmful molecules called free radicals. Free radicals are unstable molecules that can damage cells, proteins, and DNA within the body, leading to various health problems and aging. Antioxidants neutralize free radicals by donating an electron, thus preventing or minimizing their damaging effects.

Common antioxidants include:

VITAMINS:

Certain vitamins have antioxidant properties. These include vitamin C, vitamin E, and beta-carotene (a precursor to vitamin A). They are found in various fruits, vegetables, nuts, and seeds.

MINERALS:

Minerals such as selenium and manganese act as antioxidants in the body. Selenium, in particular, is essential for the proper function of antioxidant enzymes.

PHYTOCHEMICALS:

Many plant compounds, known as phytochemicals or polyphenols, have antioxidant properties. These include flavonoids (found in fruits and vegetables), resveratrol (found in red wine and grapes), and curcumin (found in turmeric).

ENZYMES:

The body produces its own antioxidant enzymes, such as superoxide dismutase (SOD), catalase, and glutathione peroxidase, to help neutralize free radicals.

Antioxidants offer several potential health benefits:

PROTECTION AGAINST OXIDATIVE STRESS:

Oxidative stress, caused by an imbalance between free radicals and antioxidants in the body, is linked to various chronic diseases, including cancer, heart disease, and neurodegenerative disorders. Antioxidants can help mitigate this stress.

ANTI-INFLAMMATORY EFFECTS:

Some antioxidants have anti-inflammatory properties, which can help reduce inflammation and the risk of inflammatory diseases.

SKIN HEALTH:

Antioxidants like vitamin C and vitamin E are commonly used in skincare products because they can protect the skin from damage caused by UV radiation and environmental pollutants.

AGING:

While aging is a natural process, oxidative stress is believed to contribute to premature aging. Antioxidants may help slow down the aging process by reducing oxidative damage to cells and tissues.

IMMUNE SUPPORT:

Antioxidants play a role in supporting the immune system by protecting immune cells from oxidative damage.

It's important to note that while antioxidants offer potential health benefits, consuming them in the form of whole foods is generally more beneficial than relying solely on supplements. A diet rich in fruits, vegetables, nuts, seeds, and whole grains provides a wide range of antioxidants along with other essential nutrients.

PHYTONUTRIENTS

PHYTONUTRIENTS

Phytonutrients, also known as phytochemicals, are naturally occurring compounds found in plants that have various health-promoting properties. These compounds are not considered essential nutrients like vitamins and minerals, but they offer a wide range of health benefits when included in your diet. Phytonutrients are responsible for the vibrant colors, flavors, and scents of many fruits, vegetables, and herbs.

FLAVONOIDS:

These are one of the most common classes of phytonutrients and include subgroups like anthocyanins (found in berries, red cabbage, and red wine), flavones (found in parsley and celery), and flavonols (found in onions and broccoli). Flavonoids have antioxidant, anti-inflammatory, and potentially anti-cancer properties.

CAROTENOIDS:

Carotenoids are responsible for the red, orange, and yellow colors in many fruits and vegetables. Beta-carotene (found in carrots), lycopene (found in tomatoes), and lutein (found in spinach) are examples of carotenoids. They have antioxidant properties and are important for eye health and immune function.

GLUCOSINOLATES:

These sulfur-containing compounds are found in cruciferous vegetables like broccoli, cauliflower, and Brussels sprouts. They may have cancer-fighting properties and contribute to the characteristic bitter taste of these vegetables.

PHENOLIC COMPOUNDS:

This category includes resveratrol (found in red grapes and wine), curcumin (found in turmeric), and ellagic acid (found in berries). Phenolic compounds have antioxidant and anti-inflammatory effects and may support heart health and reduce the risk of chronic diseases.

SAPONINS:

These are compounds found in legumes like chickpeas and lentils. They may have immune-boosting and anti-inflammatory properties.

ALLYL SULFIDES:

These compounds are found in garlic, onions, and leeks and are associated with potential cardiovascular benefits.

TERPENES:

These compounds are found in citrus fruits and are known for their aromatic qualities. They may have anti-inflammatory and antioxidant effects.

The health benefits of phytonutrients are wide-ranging and include:

ANTIOXIDANT ACTIVITY:

Many phytonutrients have strong antioxidant properties, which help protect cells from damage caused by free radicals.

ANTI-INFLAMMATORY EFFECTS:

Some phytonutrients can reduce inflammation in the body, which is linked to chronic diseases like heart disease and arthritis.

CANCER PREVENTION:

Certain phytonutrients may help prevent or slow the growth of cancer cells.

HEART HEALTH:

Phytonutrients can support heart health by reducing cholesterol levels, improving blood vessel function, and reducing the risk of blood clots.

EYE HEALTH:

Carotenoids, such as lutein and zeaxanthin, are important for maintaining good vision and reducing the risk of age-related macular degeneration.

To benefit from phytonutrients, it's important to consume a diverse range of fruits, vegetables, nuts, seeds, and whole grains in your diet. Different plant foods contain different phytonutrients, so eating a variety of these foods is the best way to ensure you get a broad spectrum of health-promoting compounds.

ESSENTIAL

FATTY ACIDS

ESSENTIAL FATTY ACIDS

Essential fatty acids (EFAs) are specific types of fats that are necessary for the proper functioning of the human body, but the body cannot produce them on its own. Therefore, they must be obtained through the diet. There are two primary types of essential fatty acids:

OMEGA-3 FATTY ACIDS:

Omega-3 fatty acids are polyunsaturated fats that are important for various bodily functions, including brain health, heart health, and reducing inflammation. The three main types of omega-3 fatty acids are:

a. **ALPHA-LINOLENIC ACID (ALA):**

This is found in plant-based sources such as flaxseeds, chia seeds, and walnuts.

b. **EICOSAPENTAENOIC ACID (EPA):**

Found in fatty fish like salmon, mackerel, and sardines, as well as fish oil supplements.

c. **DOCOSAHEXAENOIC ACID (DHA):**

Also found in fatty fish and fish oil supplements. DHA is particularly important for brain and eye health.

OMEGA-6 FATTY ACIDS:

Omega-6 fatty acids are also polyunsaturated fats, and they play a role in various bodily functions, including cell growth and inflammation response. The primary omega-6 fatty acid is linoleic acid, which is commonly found in vegetable oils (e.g., soybean oil, corn oil) and various processed foods.

CELL STRUCTURE:

They are a crucial component of cell membranes, helping to maintain their fluidity and integrity.

BRAIN FUNCTION:

Omega-3 fatty acids, especially DHA, are essential for proper brain development and function. They are particularly important during pregnancy and early childhood.

HEART HEALTH:

Omega-3s have been linked to a reduced risk of heart disease by lowering triglycerides, reducing inflammation, and improving blood vessel function.

INFLAMMATION REGULATION:

EFAs play a role in regulating inflammation in the body. Omega-3s are known for their anti-inflammatory properties.

SKIN HEALTH:

They contribute to healthy skin, hair, and nails.

HORMONE PRODUCTION:

EFAs are used in the production of hormones and other signaling molecules in the body.

It's important to maintain a balanced ratio of omega-3 to omega-6 fatty acids in the diet. In Western diets, there is often an overabundance of omega-6 fatty acids due to the prevalence of vegetable oils in processed foods. An imbalance in the ratio of these fatty acids may contribute to inflammation and various health problems. Therefore, it's recommended to include sources of omega-3s in your diet, such as fatty fish or plant-based options like flaxseeds and walnuts, to help maintain a healthy balance.

AMINO ACIDS

AMINO ACIDS

Amino acids are organic compounds that serve as the building blocks of proteins in living organisms. Proteins are essential macromolecules with a wide range of functions in the body, including structural support, enzymatic reactions, immune function, and cell signaling. Amino acids are crucial for the synthesis of these proteins and are involved in various physiological processes. There are 20 standard amino acids that are commonly found in proteins, and they can be categorized into two groups based on how the body obtains them:

ESSENTIAL AMINO ACIDS:

These amino acids cannot be synthesized by the human body and must be obtained through the diet. There are nine essential amino acids:

a. Histidine

b. Isoleucine

c. Leucine

d. Lysine

e. Methionine

f. Phenylalanine

g. Threonine

h. Tryptophan

i. Valine

These amino acids are typically found in a variety of protein-rich foods, such as meat, poultry, fish, dairy products, legumes, and some grains and nuts.

NON-ESSENTIAL AMINO ACIDS:

The body can synthesize these amino acids from other compounds, and they are not strictly required in the diet. There are 11 non-essential amino acids:

a. Alanine

b. Arginine

c. Asparagine

d. Aspartic Acid

e. Cysteine

f. Glutamine

g. Glutamic Acid

h. Glycine

i. Proline

j. Serine

k. Tyrosine

While these amino acids can be synthesized by the body, there are certain situations, such as illness or stress, where their dietary intake may become important.

Amino acids are not only critical for protein synthesis but also serve as precursors for various molecules in the body. For example, some amino acids can be converted into neurotransmitters, hormones, and metabolic intermediates.

The specific sequence and arrangement of amino acids in a protein determine its structure and function. The body uses genetic information encoded in DNA to specify the order of amino acids in a protein, and this sequence determines the protein's unique properties.

ELECTROLYTES

ELECTROLYTES

Electrolytes are electrically charged ions that play a crucial role in various physiological processes within the human body. These ions are essential for maintaining proper functioning of cells, tissues, and organs. The most common electrolytes in the human body include:

SODIUM (NA+):

Sodium is the primary extracellular cation and is essential for maintaining fluid balance, nerve function, and muscle contraction. It also plays a role in maintaining blood pressure.

POTASSIUM (K+):

Potassium is the primary intracellular cation and is vital for proper nerve and muscle function, including the heartbeat. It helps maintain the body's electrical balance.

CALCIUM (CA2+):

Calcium is essential for bone and teeth health, blood clotting, muscle contraction (including the heart), and nerve signaling.

MAGNESIUM (MG2+):

Magnesium is involved in hundreds of enzymatic reactions in the body, including those related to energy production, muscle and nerve function, and the synthesis of DNA and RNA.

CHLORIDE (CL-):

Chloride ions are often found alongside sodium in extracellular fluid and play a role in maintaining electrolyte balance, osmotic pressure, and pH balance.

BICARBONATE (HCO3-):

Bicarbonate ions are crucial for maintaining the body's acid-base balance. They help buffer acids and bases in the blood and tissues to keep pH within a narrow range.

Electrolytes are primarily found in bodily fluids like blood, plasma, and extracellular fluid. Maintaining the right balance of electrolytes is essential for various physiological functions, including:

NERVE FUNCTION:

Electrolytes are involved in transmitting electrical signals between nerve cells, allowing for communication within the nervous system.

MUSCLE CONTRACTION:

Calcium and potassium are particularly important for muscle contractions. An imbalance in these electrolytes can lead to muscle cramps and weakness.

HEART FUNCTION:

Sodium, potassium, and calcium are critical for maintaining the electrical activity of the heart. Proper electrolyte balance is essential for a regular heartbeat.

FLUID BALANCE:

Sodium and chloride help regulate the balance of fluids in and out of cells, ensuring that cells maintain the correct volume and preventing dehydration or swelling.

PH REGULATION:

Bicarbonate ions play a key role in maintaining blood pH within a narrow range, which is critical for overall metabolic function.

Electrolyte imbalances, either through excessive loss (e.g., through sweating, diarrhea, or kidney dysfunction) or excessive intake (e.g., through excessive salt consumption), can lead to health problems. Common issues associated with electrolyte imbalances include muscle cramps, irregular heart rhythms, dehydration, and fatigue. In severe cases, electrolyte imbalances can be life-threatening and require medical intervention.

To maintain proper electrolyte balance, it's important to consume a balanced diet with sufficient intake of electrolyte-containing foods and fluids. Athletes and individuals who engage in strenuous physical activity may need to pay particular attention to their electrolyte intake to replace what is lost through sweating.

CHOLINE

CHOLINE

Choline is an essential nutrient that plays a critical role in various physiological processes in the human body. It is often grouped with the B-vitamins due to its similar functions and properties. Choline is important for several reasons:

CELL MEMBRANE STRUCTURE:

Choline is a component of phospholipids, which are essential for the structure and integrity of cell membranes. Phospholipids make up the lipid bilayer that surrounds and protects cells.

NEUROTRANSMITTER SYNTHESIS:

Choline is a precursor for acetylcholine, a neurotransmitter that plays a crucial role in various nervous system functions, including muscle control, memory, and mood regulation.

BRAIN DEVELOPMENT:

Adequate choline intake during pregnancy and infancy is critical for proper brain development, including the formation of neural tube structures. Choline is also important for cognitive function throughout life.

LIVER FUNCTION:

Choline is involved in the metabolism of fat in the liver. It helps prevent the accumulation of fat in the liver, which can lead to non-alcoholic fatty liver disease (NAFLD).

METHYLATION REACTIONS:

Choline is a key source of methyl groups in the body, which are involved in numerous biochemical reactions, including DNA synthesis, detoxification, and the regulation of gene expression.

CHOLINE DEFICIENCY:

A deficiency of choline can lead to various health issues, including liver damage, muscle damage, and cognitive impairment.

Choline can be obtained through the diet and is present in various foods, including:

Eggs: Egg yolks are a particularly rich source of choline.

Meat: Chicken, beef, and pork are good sources of choline.

Fish: Fish like salmon and cod contain choline.

Dairy Products: Milk and dairy products provide choline.

Legumes: Some legumes, such as soybeans, also contain choline.

Nuts: Certain nuts, including peanuts and almonds, contain choline.

The recommended daily intake of choline can vary depending on factors such as age, sex, and life stage (e.g., pregnancy or lactation). It is important to ensure an adequate intake of choline through dietary sources or supplements if necessary, especially for individuals who may have higher requirements due to specific health conditions or life stages.

Choline is generally considered safe when consumed within recommended dietary levels. However, excessive choline intake from supplements can lead to side effects such as fishy body odor, low blood pressure, and gastrointestinal distress. It's advisable to consult with a healthcare professional before taking choline supplements, especially at high doses.

TRACE ELEMENTS

TRACE ELEMENTS

Trace elements, also known as trace minerals or micronutrients, are minerals that the human body requires in very small amounts for various physiological functions. While the body needs these minerals in smaller quantities compared to major minerals like calcium and potassium, they are still essential for maintaining good health. Trace elements play a crucial role in various biochemical and metabolic processes. Some of the most important trace elements include:

IRON (Fe):

Iron is vital for the formation of hemoglobin, which carries oxygen in the blood. Iron is also a component of myoglobin, which stores oxygen in muscle tissue. Iron deficiency can lead to anemia.

ZINC (Zn):

Zinc is involved in numerous enzymatic reactions and plays a role in immune function, wound healing, DNA synthesis, and the senses of taste and smell. It is essential for growth and development.

COPPER (Cu):

Copper is a component of enzymes involved in iron metabolism, connective tissue formation, and the production of energy. It also plays a role in maintaining healthy bones and nerves.

SELENIUM (Se):

Selenium is an antioxidant that helps protect cells from damage caused by free radicals. It is also essential for thyroid function and plays a role in the immune system.

IODINE (I):

Iodine is crucial for the synthesis of thyroid hormones, which regulate metabolism and overall growth and development. Iodine deficiency can lead to thyroid disorders.

MANGANESE (Mn):

Manganese is a cofactor for various enzymes involved in bone formation, blood clotting, and energy metabolism.

FLUORIDE (F):

Fluoride is important for dental health. It helps prevent tooth decay by strengthening tooth enamel and making it more resistant to acid erosion.

MOLYBDENUM (Mo):

Molybdenum is a cofactor for enzymes involved in the metabolism of certain amino acids and the conversion of purines into uric acid.

CHROMIUM (Cr):

Chromium plays a role in insulin action, helping to regulate blood sugar levels. It is important for carbohydrate and lipid metabolism.

COBALT (Co):

Cobalt is a component of vitamin B12 (cobalamin), which is essential for the production of red blood cells and the functioning of the nervous system.

Trace elements are typically obtained through the diet, as the body cannot produce them in sufficient quantities on its own. A balanced and varied diet that includes a wide range of foods can help ensure adequate intake of these essential trace minerals. In some cases, dietary supplements may be recommended to address specific deficiencies or meet increased requirements, especially in individuals with certain health conditions or special dietary needs.

It's important to note that while trace elements are essential, excessive intake can be harmful. Therefore, it's important to meet recommended dietary intake levels without exceeding them, as excessive intake of some trace elements can lead to toxicity and health problems.

PROBIOTICS

PROBIOTICS

Probiotics are live microorganisms, primarily bacteria and, to a lesser extent, yeast, that are beneficial for human health when consumed in adequate amounts. These "friendly" or "good" bacteria are believed to promote a healthy balance of gut microbiota, which has various positive effects on the body. Probiotics are often referred to as "live cultures."

Here are some key points about probiotics:

GUT HEALTH:

Probiotics are most commonly associated with improving gut health. They help maintain a healthy balance of microorganisms in the intestines, which is important for proper digestion, nutrient absorption, and overall digestive health.

TYPES OF PROBIOTICS:

Probiotics include various strains of bacteria, with the most common types belonging to the genera Lactobacillus and Bifidobacterium. Examples include Lactobacillus acidophilus, Bifidobacterium bifidum, and many others. Each strain may have slightly different effects on the body.

SOURCES:

Probiotics can be found in certain foods and dietary supplements. Common food sources of probiotics include yogurt, kefir, sauerkraut, kimchi, miso, and some fermented cheeses. Probiotic supplements are also widely available and may contain a combination of bacterial strains.

HEALTH BENEFITS:

Probiotics have been studied for their potential health benefits, which may include:

IMPROVED DIGESTION:

Probiotics can help with conditions like diarrhea, irritable bowel syndrome (IBS), and lactose intolerance.

ENHANCED IMMUNE FUNCTION:

A healthy gut microbiome is thought to support a strong immune system.

PREVENTION OF INFECTIONS:

Probiotics may help prevent or reduce the severity of certain infections, such as urinary tract infections and vaginal yeast infections.

REDUCED INFLAMMATION:

Some studies suggest that probiotics may help reduce inflammation in the gut and throughout the body, which is associated with various chronic diseases.

MENTAL HEALTH:

Emerging research suggests a potential link between gut health and mental health, with some evidence that probiotics may have a positive impact on mood and stress.

DOSAGE AND TIMING:

The effectiveness of probiotics can depend on factors such as the specific strains used, the dosage, and the timing of consumption. Different strains may be more effective for different conditions.

SAFETY:

In general, probiotics are considered safe for most healthy individuals. However, people with weakened immune systems or underlying health conditions should consult with a healthcare professional before taking probiotic supplements, as there may be risks associated with certain strains.

QUALITY AND STORAGE:

When choosing probiotic supplements, it's important to select reputable brands with well-documented strains and potency. Probiotic supplements should be stored as directed to maintain the viability of the live cultures.

It's essential to note that the effects of probiotics can vary from person to person, and not all probiotics are effective for all conditions. If you're considering using probiotics for a specific health concern, it's advisable to consult with a healthcare provider who can offer guidance on the most appropriate strains and dosage for your needs. Additionally, a balanced diet that includes a variety of fiber-rich foods can naturally support a healthy gut microbiome.

The End